Trim Triumph :Your Simple Roadmap to Success!"

Charles J. Hickman

INTRODUCTION

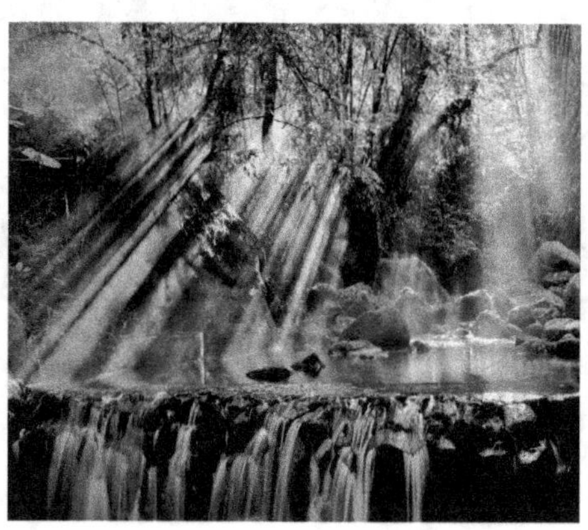

In the bustling heart of a small town, Charles J. Hickman found himself at a crossroads. A self-proclaimed lover of life, he was facing a challenge that many could relate to—a battle with unwanted cravings and the persistent struggle to lose weight. Little did he know, this personal struggle would become the catalyst for a transformative journey and the inspiration behind the book that would resonate with countless individuals seeking a path to wellness.

Charles, a man of humble beginnings, had always approached life with zest and enthusiasm. He revelled in the simple pleasures, be it the warmth of a sunrise or the comforting embrace of his favourite chair after a long day. Yet, as life unfolded, so did the demands and stresses that often accompany adulthood.

It was during a routine doctor's visit that Charles received a wake-up call. The scale revealed a number that startled him, a stark reminder of the toll his lifestyle had taken on his health. Frustration and self-reflection set in as he grappled with the reality of his situation. It was at this moment of vulnerability that Charles made a decision—to not let this setback define him but to use it as a springboard for positive change.

The journey began with introspection. Charles delved into the root of his cravings, exploring the emotional and psychological triggers that led him to indulge in unhealthy habits. This process of self-discovery became the foundation of his approach—an approach that would later form the backbone of "Trim Triumph, Lose Weight: Your Simple Roadmap to Success."

As he navigated the labyrinth of nutritional information and wellness advice, Charles realised the need for simplicity. In a world inundated with complex diets and conflicting guidelines, he sought to distil the essentials into a straightforward roadmap. This roadmap wasn't just about shedding pounds; it was about reclaiming control, fostering a positive relationship with food, and ultimately, rediscovering the joy of a healthier life.

The journey wasn't without its challenges. Charles faced setbacks, moments of doubt, and the lure of old habits. Yet, with resilience and the lessons learned along the way, he continued to refine his approach. The process became more than a physical transformation; it became a profound shift in mindset and lifestyle.

"Trim Triumph, Lose Weight" emerged as more than a guide—it became a companion for those on a similar journey. Through anecdotes, practical tips, and a touch of humour, Charles shared his experiences, making the seemingly daunting task of weight loss feel relatable and achievable. The book became a beacon for those seeking a sustainable and enjoyable path to wellness.

Charles didn't just stop at sharing his story; he became a champion for others, offering support and encouragement. He recognized that each person's journey is unique and that there is no one-size-fits-all solution. Empathy became a driving force, as he understood the struggles and celebrated the victories of those who embraced his roadmap.

In the end, Charles J. Hickman's story is not just about conquering cravings and losing weight; it's about the resilience of the human spirit, the power of simplicity, and the joy that comes from reclaiming one's health. As readers embark on this journey with him, they find not only a guide to wellness but a testament to the transformative potential within us all—a potential waiting to be unleashed on the path to a healthier, happier life.

Understanding the Origins of Cravings

Understanding the nature of cravings is essential for anyone who wants to make long-term improvements in their eating habits and overall well-being. Cravings are intense desires for a particular type of food or drink that are generally marked by their quick onset and often overwhelming nature. These cravings can be activated by a number of circumstances, including emotional states, environmental cues, social interactions, and dietary deficits.

Cravings, particularly for unhealthy foods high in fat, sugar, or salt, are well-known to be a substantial barrier to obtaining and maintaining a healthy weight. According to research, these meals can trigger brain regions involved with pleasure and reward, resulting in a loop of yearning, intake, and desire. Understanding the psychological and physiological reasons underlying cravings is critical for creating effective techniques for managing and eventually overcoming them.

Furthermore, individual variability in wanting experiences must be considered. Genetics, stress, sleep patterns, and even cultural influences can all influence the strength and frequency of cravings. Recognising and appreciating these variances is critical in developing personalised methods to desire management and weight loss goals.

We can begin to untangle the multidimensional nature of cravings by diving into their multifaceted nature, laying the way for long-term and successful weight loss attempts. Let us go on this adventure together to unravel the mystery of cravings and unlock the door to a better, more balanced lifestyle. Food cravings are a health ailment with both physical and psychological or behavioural components. Food cravings are not a problem once in a while or to a limited amount; they are readily controllable and reversed. However, if not handled, it can evolve to food addictions, which are similar to drug and alcohol addictions in nature. Obesity, diabetes, heart disease, liver disease, and some malignancies are all major problems in this situation.

This book will teach us how to deal with these desires.

CHAPTER 1

How Cravings Influence Weight Loss

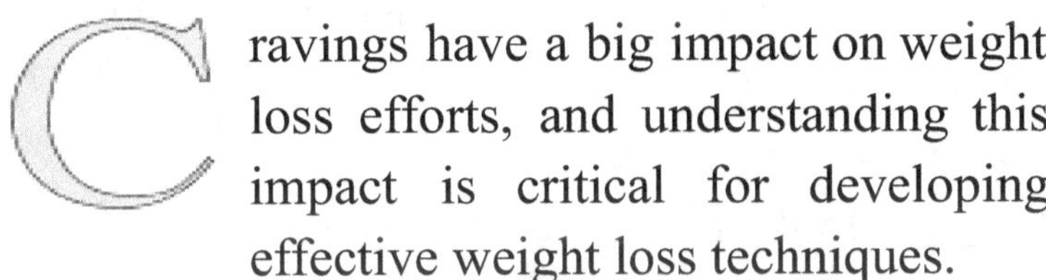

Cravings have a big impact on weight loss efforts, and understanding this impact is critical for developing effective weight loss techniques.

Physiological Consequences

1. **Consumption of Excess Calories:** Cravings frequently lead to the consumption of calorie-dense foods heavy in sweets, fats, or salts. These meals are typically deficient in key nutrients, resulting in an imbalance in calorie

intake and expenditure that can directly undermine weight loss efforts.

2. **Hormonal Imbalance:** Certain diets, particularly those high in sugar and refined carbs, can induce blood sugar rises and subsequent crashes. This might cause hormonal changes, particularly in insulin and cortisol, which can lead to increased fat storage and probable muscle loss, impeding weight loss efforts.

Psychological Consequences

1. **Disruption of Mindful Eating:** Cravings can interfere with mindfulness during meals, resulting in overeating and a lack of awareness of satiety cues. This frequently leads to a larger overall calorie intake, making it difficult to maintain the essential caloric deficit for weight loss.

2. **Emotional Eating Patterns:** Cravings are frequently associated with emotional states like tension, boredom, or grief. Emotional eating can lead to the consumption of comfort foods, which are often high in calories and low in nutritional content, interfering with weight loss goals.

Behavioural Effects

1. **Disrupted Dietary Plans:** Cravings can cause impulsive departures from planned, healthier meals, disrupting dietary adherence as well as adherence to calorie or macronutrient targets required for weight management.

2. **Reduced Motivation and Self-Efficacy:** Frequent and severe cravings can lead to feelings of guilt and diminished self-efficacy, potentially reducing motivation to stick to balanced food and exercise regimens.

<u>Social and environmental consequences</u>

1. **Social Influence and Pressure:** Cravings can be influenced by social contexts and the presence of individuals enjoying certain foods, resulting in peer pressure and subsequent indulgence in craving-inducing items.

2. **Environmental Triggers:** External cues such as ads, food availability, and even the sight or scent of specific foods can stimulate cravings, making it difficult to maintain healthy eating habits and successfully navigate weight reduction journeys.

Understanding the multiple ways in which cravings affect weight loss throws light on the need of adopting holistic techniques for desiring management while pursuing weight loss objectives. Individuals can better equip themselves to overcome these obstacles and achieve successful, long-term weight loss outcomes by addressing the physiological, psychological, and behavioural elements of cravings.

●Desiring /Cravings Management Strategies

Managing cravings effectively requires a multifaceted approach that includes mindful eating practices, detecting triggers, and substituting healthier options for harmful appetites. Let's go into the specifics.

<u>Mindful Eating Methods</u>

1. **Sensory Awareness:** Encourage people to use all of their senses while eating. This entails paying attention to the food's flavour, texture, and scent. Individuals are more likely to be satisfied by smaller servings, potentially lessening the desire to indulge in unhealthy desires.

2. **Eating Without Distractions**: Recommending that people limit their use of

distractions during meals, such as television, computers, or smartphones, allows them to establish a closer relationship with their food. This increases awareness of hunger and satiety cues, which might help you avoid impulsive, craving-driven eating.

Detecting Triggers

1.   **Emotional Awareness:** Help people understand emotional factors that contribute to cravings. Keeping a diary to document emotions and desires, assisting clients in understanding trends, and establishing alternate coping mechanisms for emotional distress can all be part of this.

2. **Environmental and Social Triggers:** Teach people how to recognise external triggers such as certain places, meals, or social circumstances that cause cravings. Once identified, individuals can avoid or plan for certain triggers, reducing their impact on craving intensity.

<u>Substituting Healthier Options for Unhealthy Cravings</u>

1. **Encourage the investigation of healthy, balanced alternatives to typical craving-inducing foods:** Substituting healthy foods like fruit, almonds, or yoghurt for packaged snacks, for example, delivers important nutrients while satisfying cravings.

2. **Portion management**: When managing urges, educate people on the necessity of portion management. Moderation is essential, and having pre-portioned healthy alternatives on hand can help prevent overeating and promote healthier eating habits.

3. **Meal Planning and Preparation:** Teach participants how to incorporate planned healthy snacks and meals into their daily routine. Having healthful options on hand minimises the

need to go for convenience foods when cravings strike, contributing to a healthier overall diet.

Individuals can get greater control over their desires by using these tactics, which will ultimately benefit their weight loss attempts. It is critical to emphasise that controlling urges is a learned skill that requires time and practise. Individuals might progressively acquire the upper hand in dealing with cravings with patience, determination, and a supportive environment, leading to improved eating patterns and successful weight management.

●Mindful/Apprehensive Eating Methods

Mindful eating entails paying more attention to what you eat and how it makes you feel. It may help minimise disordered eating behaviours and improve weight loss in addition to teaching you to discern between physical and emotional hunger.

Apprehensive eating is a fashion that helps you better manage your eating habits. It has been shown to promote weight loss, reduce binge eating, and help you feel more. Apprehensive eating ways promote a deeper, more conscious connection with the act of eating, fostering an awareness of hunger and malnutrition cues, as well as the sensitive and emotional aspects of food consumption. By rehearsing apprehensive eating, individualities can develop a healthier relationship with food, potentially reducing gluttonousness and jones . Let's explore these ways in detail.

<u>sensitive awareness</u>

1. **Savouring the Moment** :Encourage individualities to break down and savour each bite, paying attention to the flavours, textures, and aromas of the food. By fastening on sensitive exploits, individualities can decide

lower satisfaction from their reflections, potentially reducing the intensity of jones for specific, constantly hyperactive-palatable, foods.

2. **Smelling and Texture** :Emphasise the significance of smelling food fully, appreciating its texture, and being present in the act of eating. By doing so, individualities can decide further enjoyment and malnutrition from their reflections, potentially altering their relationship with food and jones .

Eating Without Distractions

1. **Apprehensive Mealtime Environment:** Encourage individualities to produce a calm, distraction-free mess terrain. This means minimising or barring distractions analogous as television, smartphones, or computers, allowing individualities to concentrate solely on the sensitive experience of eating. By doing so,

they can become more attuned to their body's hunger and wholeness cues, reducing the liability of careless gluttonousness or indulging in stewing- driven consumption.

2. **Paying Attention to Hunger and Fullness** Promote the practice of breaking periodically during a mess to check in with one's hunger situations. By tuning into the body's signals, individualities can more hand when they are satisfied, potentially reducing the liability of gorging in response to jones .

Cultivating awareness

1. **Emotional Awareness**: Encourage individualities to fete and admit their emotional countries before, during, and after eating. By rehearsing emotional awareness, individualities can develop the capacity to separate between physical hunger and emotional jones , leading

to farther purposeful, apprehensive choices in their eating habits.

2. **Gratitude and Awareness :** Explore the generality of expressing appreciativeness for the food being consumed. This involves taking a moment to consider the origins of the mess, the trouble that went into its product, and the nourishment it provides. By fostering a sense of appreciativeness and awareness, individualities can approach eating with a more positive and apprehensive mindset, potentially reducing the pull of stewing- driven consumption.

By incorporating these apprehensive eating ways into their quotidian habits, individualities can begin to cultivate a farther conscious and purposeful approach to food consumption. This can lead to a lower sense of satisfaction from reflections, better awareness of hunger and malnutrition cues, and a potentially reduced vulnerability to stewing- driven eating conduct.

Apprehensive eating is not a quick- fix result, but rather a precious skill that, when rehearsed constantly, can support individuals in making healthier, more fulfilling food choices.

Constitutionally, Apprehensive Eating Involves

• eating slowly and without distraction

• harkening to physical hunger cues andeating only until you 're full

• identifying between true hunger andnon-hunger triggers for eating

• engaging your senses by noticing colours, smells, sounds, textures, and flavours

• knowledge to manage with guilt and anxiety about food

• eating to maintain overall health and well-being

• noticing the goods food has on your heartstrings and body

• appreciating your food These goods allow you to replace automatic studies and responses with farther conscious, health- promoting responses.

Why Should You Try Apprehensive Eating?
Distractions have shifted attention down from the factual act of eating toward boxes, computers, and smartphones.

By eating mindfully, you restore your attention and slow down, making eating an intentional act instead of an automatic one.

What's more, by increasing your recognition of physical hunger and fullness cues, you can distinguish between emotional and true physical hunger .

You also increase your awareness of triggers that make you want to eat, even though you're not necessarily hungry .Knowing your triggers allows you to create a space between them and your response, giving you the time and freedom to choose how to react.

<u>Careful Eating and Weight Reduction</u>

It's notable that utmost get-healthy plans do not work in the long haul. As a matter of fact, some disquisition proposes that individualities will generally recover about a portion of the chalet pounds following 2 times and 80 of the chalet pounds following 5 times. BED, profound eating, outside endlessly eating in light of food solicitations have been connected to weight gain and recovery after fruitful weight reduction.

Constant openness to stress may likewise assume an enormous part in gorging and weight. utmost examinations concur that careful eating assists you with slipping pounds by changing your eating ways of carrying and dwindling pressure. Curiously, one inspection of 10 examinations discovered that careful eating was as important for weight reduction as normal weight reduction of 4 pounds(lb) or1.9 kilograms(kg) and further developed identity awareness, tone- acknowledgment, and tone-sympathy .

By altering the manner in which you consider food, the pessimistic sentiments that might be related with eating are superseded with awareness, working on restraint, and positive passions. While undesirable eating ways of carrying are tended to, your possibilities of long haul weight reduction achievement are expanded.

Desires are those powerful cravings for explicit food varieties that can some of the time feel like they control us more than we control them! Distinguishing triggers for food desires can be a pivotal move toward figuring out our relationship with food and pursuing better decisions. We should plunge into this exhaustively.

●Figuring out Food Desires/Identifying Triggers

Desires are the profound longings for explicit food sources, frequently high in sugar, fat, or salt. These desires can be set off by different elements, including profound, natural, and physiological signals. Understanding and recognizing these triggers can assist people with coming to informed conclusions about their dietary patterns.

<u>Recognizing Triggers</u>

1. **Close to home Triggers:** Stress, tension, fatigue, pity, and even satisfaction can set off desires. Individuals frequently go to nourishment for solace, which can prompt

explicit close to home triggers for specific food sources.

2. Ecological Triggers: Natural signs, like the sight or smell of food, promotions, or the presence of explicit food sources in the climate, can set off desires. For instance, passing by a bread kitchen or seeing a business for a most loved tidbit can set off a hankering.

3. Constant Triggers: Certain schedules and propensities can set off desires. For instance, on the off chance that somebody routinely snacks while staring at the television, the demonstration of sitting in front of the television can turn into a trigger for desires.

4. Nourishing Lacks: Once in a while, the body might desire explicit food sources because of a lack of specific supplements. For instance, wanting red meat could demonstrate a requirement for iron, while hankering chocolate could flag a requirement for magnesium.

5. **Social Triggers:** Social circumstances, like gatherings, get-togethers, or eating out with companions, can frequently set off desires. Associating with others and seeing them partake in a specific food can provoke desires for that food.

<u>Overseeing Food Desires</u>

When triggers for food desires are distinguished, overseeing them turns into the subsequent stage. A few techniques to oversee food desires include:

1. **Careful Eating:** Taking part in careful eating practices can assist people with turning out to be more mindful of their close to home and actual signs connected with food desires.

2. **Stress The executives**: Embracing pressure decreasing procedures like activity, reflection, or profound breathing can assist with overseeing desires set off by pressure.

3. **Solid Other options:** Having better choices for the food varieties that trigger desires can be helpful. For instance, subbing a sweet nibble with a piece of natural product or a small bunch of nuts.

4. **Adjusted Nourishment:** Guaranteeing that feasts are adjusted and give a blend of supplements can assist with diminishing desires brought about by dietary inadequacies.

Recognizing triggers for food desires is a fundamental stage in overseeing our dietary patterns. By perceiving the variables that lead to explicit desires, people can foster techniques to successfully address and deal with these triggers.

Keep in mind, it's vital to move toward this cycle with self-sympathy and without judgement. We as a whole have extraordinary associations with food, and understanding our triggers is a positive move toward pursuing cognizant decisions about what we eat.

I trust this reveals some insight into the subject! Assuming you have additional inquiries or need further subtleties, go ahead and inquire. Furthermore, recollect, it's OK to enjoy control — balance is critical!

•Subbing / Substituting unfortunate desires with better choices includes

Distinguishing nutritious options that can fulfil desires while adding to a fair eating regimen. By making conscious, better decisions because of desires, people can uphold their weight reduction objectives and in general prosperity.

We should jump into the subtleties of this methodology.

<u>Adjusted Other options</u>

1. **Products of the soil Replacements:** Urge people to go after leafy foods while hankering something sweet or flavorful. For instance, rather than going after a sweet treat, they could decide on a small bunch of berries, a cut apple, or carrot sticks with hummus. These choices give regular pleasantness or fulfilling smash while conveying fundamental nutrients, minerals, and fibre.

2. **Entire Grains and Vegetables:** Recommend integrating entire grains and vegetables into feasts and bites. These choices, like earthy coloured rice, quinoa, lentils, or chickpeas, offer a supplement thick, high-fibre option in contrast to handled, fatty food varieties. For example, a serving of earthy coloured rice with

blended vegetables can give a fantastic, sound choice when contrasted with handled snacks.

Segment Control

1. **Nuts and Seeds:** Nuts and seeds can act as a satisfying and supplement rich substitute for pungent, unhealthy tidbits. Notwithstanding, segment control is urgent because of their calorie thickness. Urge people to pre-segment nuts and seeds into nibble measured compartments to forestall overconsumption.

2. **Normal Nut Margarines:** Regular nut spreads, for example, almond or cashew margarine, can be a better option in contrast to spreads high in added sugars and unfortunate facts. When matched with entire grain saltines or apple cuts, they give a fantastic, supplement thick choice that can assist with suppressing desires.

Feast Arranging and Planning

1. **Protein-Stuffed Tidbits:** Empower the consideration of protein-rich bites, like Greek yoghurt, hard-bubbled eggs, or lean turkey cuts, in feast arranging. These choices can give a sensation of totality and fulfilment, possibly diminishing the probability of hankering driven nibbling.

2. **Solid Guilty pleasures:** Investigate the joining of hand crafted, better variants of liberal treats. For instance, people can explore different avenues regarding recipes for hand crafted energy bars, smoothies, or low-sugar treats utilising nutritious fixings like oats, nuts, seeds, and regular sugars like honey or dates.

By effectively searching out and embracing better options in contrast to customary hankering actuating food sources, people can reshape their relationship with food while supporting their generally speaking healthful admission. It means quite a bit to move toward this cycle with an open mentality, looking for assortment and equilibrium in the decisions made. After some time, with commitment and investigation, people can find a scope of fulfilling, better choices that line up with their weight reduction objectives and add to a seriously supporting, manageable dietary methodology.

CHAPTER 2

Underpinnings of Cravings (desires)

The underpinnings of desires are established in a complicated transaction of mental, physiological, and natural factors, all of which can add to the powerful longing for explicit food varieties or beverages. Understanding these underpinnings is vital for creating compelling systems to oversee desires and backing by and large prosperity. We should investigate the vital parts exhaustively.

Mental Underpinnings

1. **Profound Eating:** Desires frequently arise because of close to home states like pressure, fatigue, trouble, or dejection. Compelling profound associations with explicit food sources can prompt the utilisation of food as a survival technique, supporting hankering driven utilisation.

2. **Reward Pathways:** Utilisation of specific food varieties, particularly those high in fat and sugar, can actuate cerebrum areas related with delight and prize, like the limbic framework. Over the long haul, this can cause serious areas of strength to make affiliations, prompting elevated hankering reactions.

3. **Moulding and Memory:** Ecological and situational prompts, like the sight or smell of explicit food sources, can set off recollections and affiliations that lead to desires. These learned reactions can be profoundly imbued and may add to visit, deep desires.

Physiological Underpinnings

1. **Hormonal Guideline:** Desires can be affected by hormonal changes, particularly those connected with craving control and glucose guidelines. For instance, awkward nature in insulin, leptin, and ghrelin levels might affect hankering power and recurrence.

2. **Synapse Movement:** Synapses, for example, dopamine and serotonin assume a part in managing state of mind and prize. Certain food varieties can set off the arrival of these synapses, possibly adding to expanded hankering reactions.

3. **Stomach Mind Hub:** Arising research recommends that the stomach microbiota may assume a part in impacting food inclinations and desires. Irregular characteristics in stomach microscopic organisms populaces might actually affect synapse flagging and hunger guidelines, adding to desires for explicit food varieties.

Natural and Sociocultural Underpinnings

1. **Food Accessibility and Openness:** The universality of handled, unhealthy food varieties in present day conditions can enhance desires. Simple admittance to these food sources can pursue them as the go-to decision when desires strike, sustaining undesirable eating designs.

2. **Social Impacts:** Social circumstances, peer pressure, and social practices can impact

desires. For example, the presence of others eating specific food sources can set off desires, while accepted practices and customs might direct unambiguous hankering instigating food sources.

●Emotional Eating / Mental Underpinnings and its Impact on Weight Loss

1. **Mental Inclinations:** Mental cycles, for example, particular consideration and memory predispositions, can impact the discernment and notability of explicit food varieties, possibly heightening desires for those food sources.

2. **Hope and Expectation:** The simple expectation of eating a particular food can set off desires. Mental cycles connected with remuneration expectation and acquainted learning add to the enhancement of desires.

Understanding the multi-layered underpinnings of desires reveals insight into the complicated idea of these encounters. By perceiving the mental, physiological, and natural variables at play, people can foster a more nuanced, far reaching way to deal with overseeing and answering desires. By tending to these different underpinnings, people can pursue building procedures that include profound guidelines, adjusted sustenance, and mental social methods, eventually supporting better eating ways of behaving and prosperity.

Close to home eating, frequently characterised as the utilisation of food because of profound signals instead of physiological craving, can significantly affect weight on the board and in general prosperity. Figuring out the elements of profound eating, its triggers, and its ramifications is essential for creating procedures to address this way of behaving. We should jump into the subtleties.

Figuring out Close to home Eating

1. **Profound Triggers:** Close to home eating is many times incited by a scope of feelings like pressure, weariness, trouble, dejection, uneasiness, or even satisfaction. These feelings can act as powerful signals that trigger a craving for explicit food varieties, normally those high in sugar, fat, or salt, for looking for solace or help.

2. **Survival strategy:** For some people, close to home eating fills in as a way of dealing with stress to oversee and lighten trouble. Eating specific food varieties can prompt brief sensations of delight and interruption, offering a method for relieving close to home distress temporarily.

3. **Detached Eating:** Close to home eating is regularly connected with careless, disengaged eating, where people might devour food quickly and in huge amounts, frequently without enrolling sensations of satiety. This absence of mindfulness

can prompt unreasonable calorie admission and block weight the board endeavours.

Influence on Weight reduction

1. **Caloric Excess:** Profound eating can bring about the utilisation of overabundant calories past what the body needs for energy, prompting a caloric excess. After some time, this excess adds to weight gain and can hinder progress towards weight reduction objectives.

2. **Supplement Unfortunate Decisions:** Close to home eating frequently includes the determination of exceptionally tasteful, handled, and calorie-thick food sources, commonly ailing in fundamental supplements. This can prompt imbalanced sustenance, possibly influencing generally wellbeing and prosperity.

3. **Pattern of Responsibility and Disgrace:** Following episodes of close to home eating, people might encounter sensations of culpability, disgrace, or lament, particularly on the off chance that they

see the way of behaving as a difficulty to their weight reduction venture. This close to home reaction might possibly set off additional episodes of profound eating, propagating an unsafe cycle.

Strategies for Addressing Emotional Eating

1. **Profound Mindfulness:** Empowering people to develop close to home mindfulness can help them perceive and recognize their profound triggers. This includes building the ability to recognize feelings and separate between obvious appetite and close to home desires.

2. **Elective Ways of dealing with hardship or stress:** Supporting people in creating elective, non-food-related techniques to deal with feelings is fundamental. This can include taking part in exercises, for example, work out, care works on, journaling, or looking for social help to address profound pain.

3. **Careful Eating Works on:** Integrating careful eating strategies, for example, focusing on actual

yearning prompts and enjoying the tactile experience of food, can assist people with turning out to be more receptive to their body's necessities and diminish hasty, sincerely determined eating.

By perceiving the effect of profound eating on the weight of the executives and prosperity, people can start to foster a more careful, purposeful way to deal with tending to close to home triggers and reshaping their relationship with food. Through a mix of profound mindfulness, elective survival strategies, and careful eating rehearsals, people can develop a better, more adjusted way to deal with feelings and support fruitful weight the board.

•Cognitive Behavioural Approaches to Craving Control

Individuals seeking to conquer cravings and build improved eating habits can benefit from cognitive behavioural techniques. These research-based strategies concentrate on recognising and changing cognitive patterns, beliefs, and behaviours that contribute to craving-driven consuming. Individuals can obtain a better knowledge and control over their urges by addressing cognitive and behavioural components. Let's take a closer look at these approaches.

Restructuring of the Mind

1. **Identifying Triggering Thoughts:** Encourage people to recognise and capture thoughts and beliefs that arise when they are seeking something. This can include recognising automatic, tempting ideas like "I need to eat this right now," or rationalising views like "I've had a rough day, so I deserve this."

2. **Unhelpful Thoughts Can Be Challenged:** Once identified, individuals can concentrate on questioning these automatic thoughts and beliefs. This may entail challenging the facts underlying these beliefs, examining alternate interpretations, and reframing them in a more balanced, rational manner.

Techniques Based on Mindfulness

1. **Thought Observation:** Helping people notice their ideas and urges without judgement can help them establish space between their thoughts and subsequent actions. Individuals can lessen sensitivity and impulsive responses to cravings by recognising the ephemeral nature of thoughts.

2. **Introducing people to the concept of "urge surfing,"** a mindfulness practice that involves riding out the wave of a want without acting on it. This method encourages acceptance of the urge while allowing it to pass without giving in to it.

Behavioural Techniques

1. **Developing Alternative Coping abilities:** Encouraging people to develop non-food-related coping abilities to deal with emotional pain and discomfort might help divert behaviour away from craving-driven consumption. This could include

physical activity, relaxation techniques, or seeking social support.

2. **Exposure and Response Prevention:** Exposing individuals to desire-inducing stimuli gradually while refusing to act on the craving can help desensitise and lessen the severity of cravings over time. This method entails acknowledging the impulse without succumbing to it.

Prevention of Relapse

1. **Identifying High-Risk scenarios:** Assisting clients in recognising high-risk scenarios, such as social events, emotional distress, or specific environmental cues, that may trigger or aggravate cravings.

2. **Creating Coping Plans:** Working with individuals to create specific, proactive techniques for dealing with high-risk circumstances, such as practising alternate responses and creating a strategy to navigate these settings without succumbing to cravings.

Self-Awareness and Self-Monitoring

1. **Keeping a Craving Diary:** Encourage people to keep a craving diary in order to note the onset, intensity, and conditions around cravings. This can provide useful insights into patterns and triggers, allowing for more tailored intervention techniques.

2. **Increasing Self-Awareness:** Increasing self-awareness and mindfulness of eating behaviours, emotions, and mental patterns. This technique helps people recognise their interior experiences and make more deliberate, balanced choices in response to urges.

Individuals might begin to gain a deeper awareness of their urges and constructive abilities to control and conquer them by adding cognitive behavioural techniques into their everyday routines. Individuals can obtain useful tools to remodel their connection with food by addressing the cognitive, emotional, and behavioural components of cravings, ultimately enabling long-term, sustainable behaviour change

CHAPTER 3

Nutritional Aspect

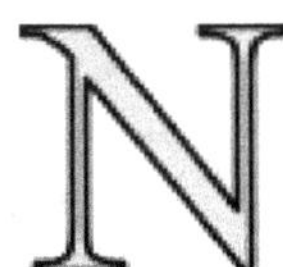

N

utritional considerations are critical in controlling cravings and assisting with weight loss efforts. Individuals can make informed choices to limit cravings and create a balanced, nourishing diet by understanding the impact of macronutrients, nutrient density, and meal composition. Let's get

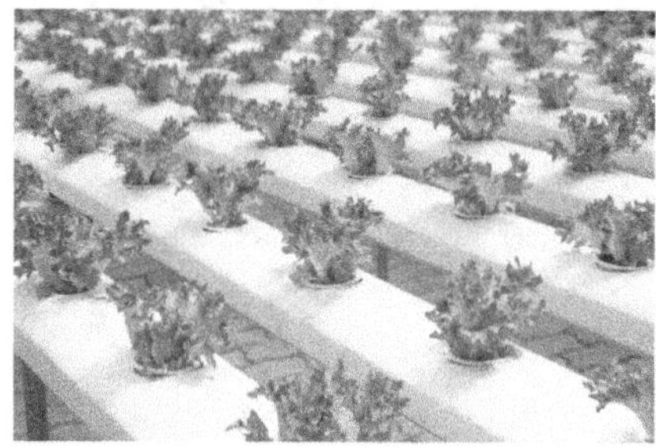

into the specifics of these dietary considerations.

●Macronutrient Balance

1. **Protein-Rich Foods:** Including lean proteins in meals and snacks might increase fullness and satiety, thus lowering the intensity and frequency of cravings. Protein-rich diets can help manage appetite and stabilise blood sugar levels, reducing cravings for high-carbohydrate, highly processed foods.

2. **Complex carbs:** Stress the need of including complex carbs into the diet, such as whole grains, legumes, and vegetables. These meals give continuous energy and fibre, which helps to maintain stable blood sugar levels and reduces the likelihood of fast changes, which can induce cravings.

3. **Healthy Fats:** Including sources of healthy fats in your diet, such as avocados, nuts, seeds, and olive oil, will help you feel satisfied and reduce cravings. When included in meals and snacks, healthy fats aid in nutrient absorption and can offer a feeling of fullness.

Foods Rich in Nutrients

1. **Micronutrient-Rich Foods:** Promoting the consumption of foods high in vital vitamins and minerals will help to improve overall health and possibly lessen cravings caused by nutrient deficits. Incorporate a variety of colourful fruits and

vegetables, as well as calcium, iron, and zinc sources.

2. **Fibre-Rich Foods:** Fibre-rich foods, such as fruits, vegetables, whole grains, and legumes, promote a feeling of fullness while also contributing to digestive health.

This can lead to more prolonged energy levels and may minimise cravings for low-nutrient, quick-fix items.

3. **Hydration:** Encouraging proper fluid intake, usually from water, promotes overall hydration and can aid with desire management. Dehydration can cause hunger, which can lead to unnecessary snacking and craving-driven eating.

Composition of Meals

1. **Regular, Balanced Meals:** Encourage people to prioritise regular, balanced meals with a variety of macronutrients. This can help to stabilise blood

sugar levels, lessen the chance of intense hunger, and potentially reduce the severity of cravings.

2. **Mindful Snacking:** Encourages the consumption of healthful, portion-controlled snacks that contain a variety of macronutrients. This strategy can help prevent energy dips between meals and lower the chance of impulsive, craving-driven snacking.

Taking Care of Nutrient Deficiencies

1. **Individualised Nutrition:** Recognising and addressing individual dietary requirements is critical for desire management. Working with a healthcare professional or certified dietitian, for example, to detect and correct any deficiencies such as iron, magnesium, or vitamin D can improve general well-being and potentially lower craving intensity.

2.**Supplementation when Necessary:** Supplementation may be necessary in cases with verified nutrient deficits. Collaboration with healthcare specialists to meet particular nutrient demands can help with desire management and general wellness.

Individuals can make informed decisions to promote a balanced, nourishing diet that may help regulate cravings, stabilise energy levels, and assist to successful long-term weight management by taking these nutritional concerns into mind. This approach promotes a holistic knowledge of the role nutrition plays in desire management and general well-being.

Macronutrient Balance to Control Cravings

Balancing macronutrients, including protein, carbs, and fats, is important for managing cravings and promoting general well-being. Each macronutrient has a distinct effect on appetite, blood sugar levels, and satiety, all of which can influence the strength and frequency of cravings. Let's take a closer look at how balancing macronutrients can help you control your cravings.

Satiety and Appetite Regulation Protein

1. **Protein-rich foods** have a high satiety value, which means they can help people feel fuller for longer periods of time, potentially lowering the likelihood of experiencing acute hunger and subsequent cravings.

2. **Protein aids in the regulation of appetite hormones** such as ghrelin and peptide YY, which can alter sensations of hunger and satiety. As a result, adequate protein consumption can help to regulate appetite and potentially minimise cravings caused by acute hunger.

3. **Metabolic Advantage:** Protein has a larger thermic effect of food (TEF) than carbohydrates or lipids. This means that the body expends more energy digesting and metabolising protein, which may aid in weight loss and contribute to more stable energy levels.

Complex Carbohydrates for Long-Term Energy and Blood Sugar Control

1. **prolonged Energy Release:** Whole grains, legumes, and vegetables contain complex carbs, which give a slow and prolonged release of glucose into the bloodstream. This slow energy release can help keep energy levels consistent and lessen the chance of abrupt blood sugar changes, which can induce cravings.

2. **Fibre Content:** Complex carbohydrates are frequently high in dietary fibre, which promotes satiety and digestive health. Fibre might help people feel content after a meal, potentially reducing cravings for between-meal snacking.

3. **Complex carbs** can help prevent the rapid increases and subsequent dips in blood sugar that can contribute to desires for quick-fix, high-sugar foods by supporting stable blood sugar levels.

Satiety and Flavour Satisfaction from Healthy Fats

1. **Satiety and Hormonal Regulation:** Including healthy fats, such as those found in nuts, seeds,

avocados, and olive oil, will help you feel full and satisfied. Furthermore, some fatty acids are involved in hormone control and signalling, which may influence hunger and desires.

2. **Flavour and contentment:** Fats contribute to the sensory experience of food and can improve flavour and contentment. This can result in a more robust and satisfying eating experience, which may reduce the urge for more, craving-driven consumption.

Appetite Control and Sustained Energy with Balanced Meal Composition

1. **Macronutrient-Rich Meals:** Promote meal composition that includes a balance of protein, complex carbs, and healthy fats. This technique can help to maintain energy levels and create a sense of fullness and pleasure, which may help to reduce cravings between meals.

2. **Portion Control:** Stress the need of balanced portion sizes in maintaining adequate macronutrient

intake without overconsumption. Overeating can cause distorted hunger and satiety signals, potentially contributing to cravings in the future.

Incorporating a diverse range of macronutrients into meals and snacks increases physiological and hormonal control, long-term energy, and a sense of fullness and satisfaction. Individuals can assist regulate their appetite, stabilise their energy levels, and potentially lessen the severity and frequency of cravings by taking this strategy, which supports general well-being and effective weight management efforts.

●Nutrient-Dense Foods to Satisfy Cravings

Incorporating nutrient-dense foods into your diet not only delivers necessary vitamins and minerals, but it can also help with cravings and overall well-being. Nutrient-dense meals provide a wide range of nutrients in relation to their calorie level, making them excellent alternatives for desire management. Let's look at some nutrient-dense foods that can help fulfil cravings while also supporting a healthy diet.

Berries and fruits

1. **Berries:** Blueberries, strawberries, and raspberries are high in antioxidants and fibre, and they have a natural sweetness and delicious texture. These foods can satisfy a sweet tooth without containing the added sugars present in many packaged snacks.

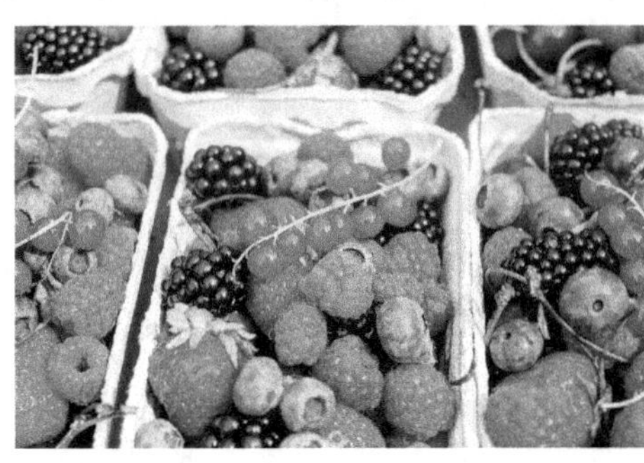

2. **Apples and pears** have a delicious crunch and are strong in fibre, which helps to induce a feeling of fullness. Fruit's natural sugars can help satisfy sweet cravings while also supplying critical nutrients.

Vegetables

1. **Crunchy Vegetables:** Carrots, celery, and bell peppers are examples of crunchy vegetables that can satisfy appetites for a crunchy, salty snack. Combining these vegetables with a nutritious dip like hummus or guacamole adds healthy fats and nutritional value.

2. **Leafy Greens:** Nutrient-dense greens such as spinach, kale and Swiss chard are adaptable and may be used in a variety of dishes. Their high fibre content can aid with satiety and desire management.

Foods High in Protein

1. **Lean Meats:** High-quality protein sources such as chicken, turkey, and lean cuts of beef can help induce a feeling of fullness and pleasure after a meal.

2. **Fatty fish** such as salmon, mackerel, and sardines include omega-3 fatty acids, which promote heart health and can help lower cravings for high-fat, less nutritional foods.

Seeds and nuts

1. **Almonds:** High in healthy fats, fibre, and protein, almonds are a filling and nutrient-dense snack. They can aid in the reduction of cravings for less nutritional, high-calorie snacks.

2. **Chia Seeds:** Rich in fibre and healthy fats, these tiny seeds can be added to yoghurt, smoothies or muesli to boost fullness and encourage satiety.

Yoghurt from Greece

1. **Yoghurt with Probiotics:** Greek yoghurt has a creamy, pleasant texture as well as probiotics, protein, and calcium. As a nutritious, craving-satisfying snack, top with fresh fruit or a small quantity of honey.

Complete Grains

1. **Quinoa:** High in protein and fibre, this nutrient-dense grain provides a feeling of fullness

and contentment. It can serve as a foundation for bowls, salads, or as a side dish.

2. **Oats:** High in fibre and recognised for their warming properties, oats can aid in the management of cravings for high-sugar, less nutritional comfort foods.

Individuals can fulfil cravings while also supporting their total nutritional intake by integrating these nutrient-dense items into meals and snacks. These selections contain necessary nutrients, increase satiety, and can aid in the management of cravings, all of which contribute to a well-balanced, healthy diet.

CHAPTER 4

Changes in Lifestyle

Lifestyle changes are critical in controlling cravings, assisting with weight loss, and increasing general well-being. Adopting a holistic strategy that includes physical activity, stress management, sleep hygiene, and social relationships can all help to promote healthy habits and resilience in the face of cravings. Let's go into the specifics of lifestyle changes that can help with desire management and establishing a healthy lifestyle.

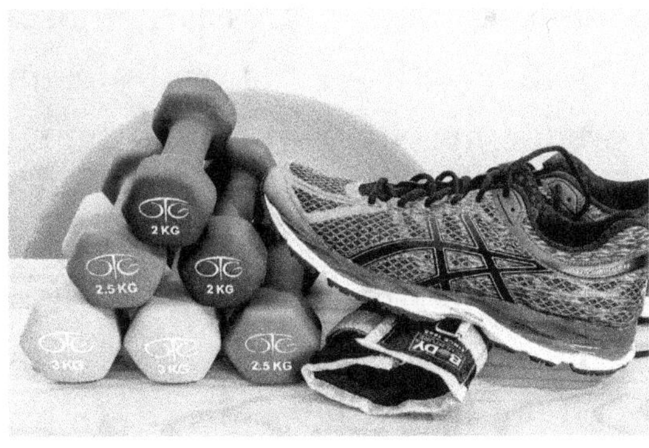

Exercise on a regular basis

1. **Regular physical activity**, such as aerobic exercise,

weight training, or other forms of movement, can help regulate appetite, enhance mood, and relieve stress, reducing the likelihood of succumbing to craving-driven snacking.

2. **Mind-Body Practises:** Trying out mind-body practises like yoga, tai chi, or meditation might help people become more aware of their bodily sensations and hunger cues, potentially lowering impulsive, craving-driven eating.

Stress Reduction

1. **Stress-Relief Techniques:** Stress-reduction approaches such as deep breathing exercises, mindfulness meditation, or progressive muscle relaxation can help with emotional eating management by reducing stress-induced hunger cues.

2. **Time Management and limits:** Having realistic expectations, prioritising self-care, and establishing healthy limits can all help to reduce stress, resulting in more balanced and mindful eating habits.

Hygiene of Sleep

1. **Adequate and Restorative Sleep:** Prioritising adequate and restorative sleep promotes general well-being and can aid in the regulation of appetite-regulating hormones, thus reducing vulnerability to energy- and craving-related imbalances.

2. **Consistent Sleep Schedule:** Having consistent sleep and wake periods will help you have more energy and be less susceptible to cravings caused by weariness or irregular sleeping habits.

Relationships and social support

1. **Create a Supportive Network:** Developing strong social ties and seeking support from friends, family, or community groups can provide emotional reinforcement and healthy coping methods, reducing the influence of emotional eating triggers.

2. **Engaging in non-food-related social activities** might contribute to a wider range of experiences

and lessen dependency on food-related socialising, thus decreasing craving-associated eating behaviours.

Environmental Improvements

1. **Healthy Food Environment:** Creating and maintaining a healthy eating environment, such as keeping nutrient-dense snacks readily available and minimising the presence of highly processed, high-calorie items, can affect eating behaviours and limit temptation.

Incorporating physical exercise into daily routines, such as taking active breaks during sedentary hours or choosing active transportation, can contribute to a more dynamic, health-supportive lifestyle.Individuals can develop a supporting framework to manage cravings, promote healthy dietary habits, and enhance general well-being by adopting these lifestyle changes. These comprehensive changes contribute to a more balanced and fulfilled existence, ultimately assisting individuals in navigating wanting triggers and making long-term, health-promoting decisions.

●Including Regular Exercise in Your Routine to Combat Cravings

Regular exercise is a great method for combating cravings, encouraging weight loss, and improving general well-being. Physical activity helps with hunger control, mood enhancement, and stress release, all of which lead to a lower susceptibility to cravings. Let's look at how regular exercise can be a helpful approach for combating cravings.

<u>Appetite Control</u>

1. **Hormonal Regulation:** Physical exercise can have a positive impact on appetite-regulating hormones including ghrelin and peptide YY, which influence hunger and satiety. This can assist individuals in achieving

a better balance in their eating habits and decreasing the risk of extreme cravings.

2. **Blood Sugar Control:** Exercise might help with blood sugar balance, potentially lowering the chance of fast blood sugar changes, which can lead to cravings for high-sugar, less nutritional foods.

3. **Metabolic Support:** Regular physical activity might help with metabolic health by improving energy utilisation and potentially lowering the intensity of hunger and cravings.

Stress Reduction and Mood Enhancement

1. **Endorphin Release:** Exercise causes endorphins to be released, which can improve mood and generate a sense of well-being. Reduced emotional eating triggers and reliance on comfort foods in reaction to stress or negative emotions can be attributed to improved emotional state.

2. **Stress Reduction:** Physical activity can assist to buffer the impact of emotional distress and lessen the incidence of stress-induced cravings. Exercise can help you cope with stress and reduce your dependency on food as a coping technique.

Increased Resilience and Distraction

1. **Cognitive Distraction:** Physical exercise provides a cognitive distraction from cravings, helping people to shift their concentration and attention away from food-related wants.

2. **Increased Resilience:** Regular exercise can help people build mental and emotional resilience, which can help them manage cravings and make more conscious, health-promoting decisions in response to food temptations.

Craving Control and Energy Balance

1. **Caloric Expenditure:** Exercise contributes to overall energy balance, allowing individuals to develop a higher calorie deficit or maintain energy balance, which can influence appetite regulation and lessen yearning frequency.

2. **Satiety Support:** Physical activity can contribute to a sense of physical exhaustion and satiety, potentially lessening the severity of cravings, particularly for high-calorie, energy-dense foods.

Incorporating regular exercise into one's regimen promotes a balanced approach to desire management, overall well-being, and weight loss success. Individuals can establish a more resilient, health-supportive lifestyle while aiming to make long-term, beneficial lifestyle changes by embracing physical activity as a strategy for combating cravings.

●Stress Management as a Priority for Better Craving Control

Stress management should be prioritised for better desire control and general well-being. Stress has a substantial impact on eating habits, leading to increased cravings for comfort foods, sugary snacks, and high-fat desserts. Individuals can lessen the intensity and frequency of cravings by effectively managing stress, making it simpler to maintain a balanced, health-supportive diet. Let's go into the specifics of how prioritising stress management helps with craving control.

The Influence of Stress on Cravings

1. **Hormonal Influence:** Stress causes the hormone cortisol, sometimes known as the stress hormone, to be released. Cortisol levels that are elevated can stimulate hunger, especially for high-calorie, sugar-rich foods, and cause intense cravings.

2. **Emotional Eating Patterns:** Stress can lead to emotional eating, in which people turn to food to cope with bad emotions. Cravings during stressful times are frequently motivated by a need for comfort and relief.

3. **Reward Pathways:** Stress can disrupt the brain's reward pathways, increasing the craving for fatty, enjoyable foods. During stressful times, these appetites function as a form of self-soothing.

Prioritising Stress Management Strategies

1. **Mindfulness and Relaxation Techniques:** Mindfulness meditation, deep breathing exercises, or progressive muscle relaxation can help people manage stress and lower the risk of cravings caused by stress.

2. **Physical Activity as a Stress Reduction approach:** Regular physical activity is a

powerful stress-reduction approach, improving mood enhancement and minimising the impact of stress on eating behaviours.

3. **Healthy Coping Mechanisms:** Promoting non-food-related stress-relief practices such as journaling, spending time in nature, or seeking social support might help to reduce dependency on food as a major coping method during stressful times.

Social Support and Emotional Support

1. **Seeking Emotional Reinforcement:** Making and maintaining healthy social connections can provide emotional reinforcement and help people manage stress, lowering the chance of emotional eating triggers.

2. **Engaging in non-food-related social activities**, such as sports, cultural events, or

hobbies, can provide a varied range of experiences and lessen reliance on food-related socialising.

Boundaries and Self-Care

1. **Having Realistic Expectations:** Having realistic expectations and creating appropriate boundaries can help to reduce the influence of stress on eating behaviours, reducing the chance of craving-driven consumption.

2. **Prioritising Self-Care Practises:** Prioritising self-care practices such as appropriate sleep, healthy nutrition, and participating in relaxing activities can boost general well-being and resilience in the face of stress-induced cravings.

Stress management, when prioritised as part of a comprehensive lifestyle strategy, can have a substantial impact on desire control and good eating behaviours. Individuals can lessen the influence of stress on their eating patterns by using effective stress management practices and developing a supportive environment, ultimately contributing to improved overall well-being and successful weight management efforts.

CHAPTER 5

Seeking Assistance

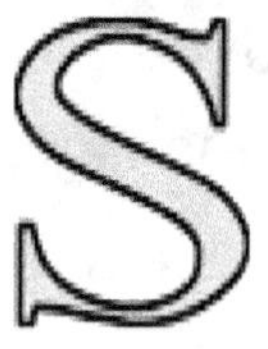

eeking help is critical in managing cravings, especially when attempting to make behavioural adjustments linked to food habits and overall well-being. Support can take many forms, including social, emotional, and professional help, all of which contribute to a more resilient, health-promoting approach to resolving cravings and developing balanced food habits. Let's go into the specifics of how seeking help might help you manage urges and live a better lifestyle.

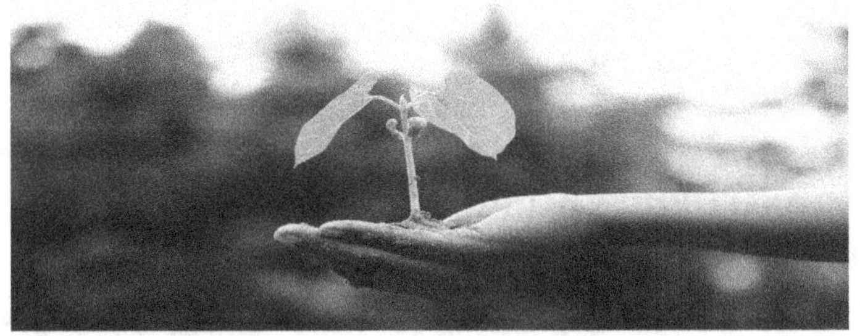

<u>Social Assistance</u>

1. **Emotional Reinforcement:** Emotional reinforcement and understanding are provided by positive social connections such as friends, family members, or support groups. These interactions provide encouragement and help strengthen a person's resilience in the face of desire cues.

2. **Accountability and Motivation:** Social networks can provide constant encouragement and affirmation as individuals struggle to manage cravings and make health-supportive decisions.

Professional Counselling and Guidance

1. **Nutritional Counselling:** Working with a certified dietitian or nutritionist can help you handle cravings, balance macronutrients, and make healthy eating choices.

2. **Therapeutic Support:** Seeking counselling or therapy, especially cognitive behavioural therapy (CBT), can help address emotional eating triggers and provide effective techniques for craving management.

Support Groups and Peer Support Networks

1. **Shared Experiences:** Connecting with others who have gone through similar experiences with cravings can create a sense of community and normalisation, lowering

feelings of isolation and promoting healthy, supportive behaviours.

2. **Skill exchanging:** Support groups can provide a forum for exchanging coping tactics and effective craving-management strategies, as well as build an environment of mutual learning and growth.

Educational Materials

1. **Information Access:** Using trustworthy educational materials, such as books, podcasts, or online forums, can provide valuable insights into regulating urges and making healthy choices, enabling continual learning and informed decision-making.

2. **Attending professional workshops and seminars** offered by healthcare professionals or experts in nutrition and behavioural psychology can provide individuals with evidence-based solutions for desire management.

Family and Household Assistance

1. **Family Nutrition:** Involving family members in healthy meal planning and nutritional cooking can foster an environment that encourages balanced dietary choices, reducing dependency on craving-inducing, convenience items.

2. **Mindful Eating Practices:** Engaging in mindful eating practises as a family, such as sharing meals and encouraging a positive, nonjudgmental approach to food, can help to create a health-supportive atmosphere.

Individuals can improve their ability to manage cravings, make healthy choices, and develop resilience in the face of craving cues by actively seeking various sorts of help. Creating a network of support, whether through social ties, professional advice, or educational resources, adds to a more complete approach to desire management and promoting a balanced, healthful lifestyle.

●Creating a Helpful Network

Having a supporting network might help you manage urges and make healthy nutritional choices. A supportive network can offer encouragement, accountability, and helpful tools, resulting in a more resilient, health-promoting approach to resolving cravings and promoting balanced eating habits. Let's go into the specifics of creating a supportive network and how it affects craving management and promoting a healthier lifestyle.

Emotional Support and Understanding

1. **Building and cultivating relationships** with friends, family members, or support groups

provides emotional reinforcement and understanding. These interactions provide encouragement and help strengthen a person's resilience in the face of desire cues.

2. Affirmation and Validation: Positive social interactions can provide affirmation and validation, alleviating feelings of isolation and self-doubt and promoting a more balanced, health-promoting mindset.

Motivation and Accountability

1. **Affirmation and Encouragement:** Supportive networks can act as sources of accountability, offering continuing encouragement and inspiration as individuals seek to manage cravings and make healthy choices.

2. **Shared Experiences:** Sharing experiences within a supportive network can build a sense

of belonging and motivation by validating problems and triumphs connected to desire management and adopting health-promoting choices.

Coping Techniques and Strategies

1. **Exchanging Skills:** Supportive networks provide essential platforms for exchanging coping skills and effective craving-management tactics, as well as establishing an environment of mutual learning and growth.

2. **Resource Exchange:** Members of a network can contribute and receive resources such as educational materials, recommended professionals, and evidence-based desire management practises.

Encouragement and support from peers

1. **Normalisation:** Interacting with others who have had similar experiences with desire management can create a sense of normalcy, lowering feelings of guilt or loneliness and strengthening health-promoting behaviours.

2. **Mutual Encouragement:** When confronted with appetite triggers, exchanging mutual encouragement within a supportive network can strengthen the pursuit of healthy eating habits and contribute to a resilient attitude.

Nutritional Choices Must Be Balanced

1. **Shared Meal Experiences:** Participating in shared meal experiences within a supportive network can provide opportunity for balanced, nutritious eating practises as well as foster a positive, supportive attitude towards food choices.

2. Nutritionally Supportive Environment: Whether among friends, family members, or peers, supportive networks can build a nutritionally friendly environment that fosters healthful, balanced dietary habits and less reliance on craving-inducing, convenience foods.

Developing a supportive network of positive social connections, shared experiences, and resource sharing can have a substantial impact on an individual's capacity to manage cravings, make healthy choices, and develop resilience in the face of craving triggers. Individuals can acquire tools and information that improve their capacity to make healthy choices and control urges effectively by actively cultivating supportive relationships and engaging with peer communities.

•Professional Counselling and Guidance for Overcoming Cravings

Seeking expert advice and counselling might help you overcome cravings and build healthier eating habits. Registered dietitians, nutritionists, and therapists, for example, can provide evidence-based techniques and therapeutic assistance to address the psychological, emotional, and behavioural aspects of desire management. Let's go into the specifics of seeking expert help and counselling to conquer urges.

Nutritional Advice

1. **Individualised Nutrition Plans:** Working with a certified dietitian or nutritionist allows individuals to obtain personalised nutrition advice tailored to their specific needs, such as strategies for addressing cravings and making health-supportive dietary choices.

2. **Macronutrient Balancing:** Nutritionists may offer expert advice on balancing macronutrients and optimising meal compositions to enhance satiety, support energy levels, and lower the chance of extreme cravings.

<u>CBT stands for Cognitive Behavioural Therapy.</u>

1. **Recognising and Addressing Emotional Eating Triggers:** CBT-trained therapists can give helpful techniques for recognising and addressing emotional eating triggers, cognitive restructuring of habitual thinking related to cravings, and the development of healthier coping skills.

2. **Skill Development:** CBT therapists provide skill-development tools to manage stress, emotional distress, and impulsive behaviours,

assisting clients in making purposeful, health-promoting choices in response to desired triggers.

Assessment of Nutrient Deficiency

1. **Identifying Nutrient Gaps:** Nutritionists can conduct assessments to identify potential nutrient deficiencies that may contribute to severe cravings, and then provide tailored methods to correct these gaps.

2. **Nutritional Supplementation:** In cases of verified nutrient deficiencies, licensed dietitians and nutritionists can provide advice on appropriate nutritional supplementation to improve general well-being and lessen the impact of deficiencies on cravings.

Emotional Eating Support

1. **Therapeutic Support:** Emotional eating and disordered eating therapists can give a helpful therapeutic setting in which to explore underlying emotional causes and establish healthier, more balanced eating patterns.

2. **Behavioural techniques:** Therapists provide evidence-based behavioural techniques and tools for controlling emotional eating behaviours as well as lowering the influence of chronic stress on craving-driven consumption.

Mindful Eating Techniques

1. **Cultivating Awareness:** Professionals can help people develop mindful eating strategies, which promote present-moment awareness during meals and snacks and can help minimise impulsive, craving-driven eating.

2. **Sensory-Based Eating:** Therapists and nutritionists can teach clients sensory-based

eating exercises to help them obtain enjoyment from meals, potentially lessening the severity of cravings.

<u>Resources and Education</u>

1.   **Access to Educational Materials:** Professionals can provide clients with access to evidence-based resources, educational materials, and credible sources of information to help them gain a deeper understanding of desire management and healthy dietary choices.
2. **Workshop and Seminar Recommendation:** Professionals might offer workshops or seminars on desire management, balanced eating, and behaviour change to provide extra learning opportunities.

Individuals can have access to a plethora of tools and evidence-based strategies for regulating cravings, building healthier eating habits, and fostering resilience in the face of craving cues by seeking help and counselling from competent specialists. Professional assistance can have a major impact on an individual's capacity to make long-term, health-promoting decisions and overcome cravings and emotional eating difficulties.

CHAPTER 6

Sustainability

In the context of healthy eating and desire management, sustainability refers to the development of long-term, balanced dietary habits and coping mechanisms that can be maintained consistently over time. A sustainable strategy addresses long-term behaviour change, desire resilience, and the continual integration of health-promoting practices into daily life. Let's look at the specifics of sustainability in terms of craving management and promoting a healthy lifestyle.

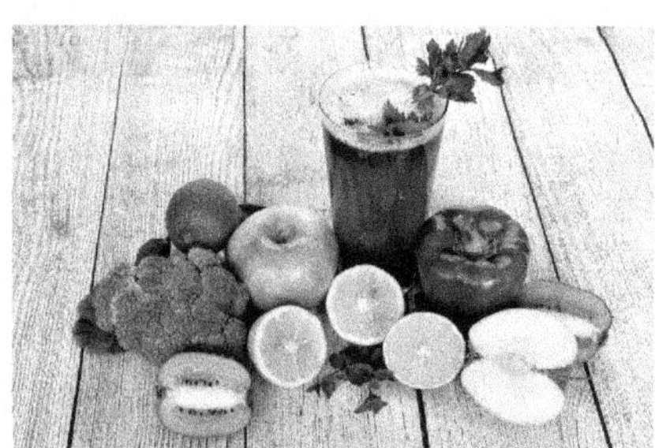

Developing Healthy Eating Habits

1. **Long-Term Mindset:** Rather than focusing on short-term, restrictive measures, a sustainable strategy emphasises the development of balanced eating patterns and coping techniques that can be continuously maintained over time.

2. **Flexible, Inclusive Approach:** A flexible, inclusive approach to food allows for occasional indulgences and emphasises moderation rather than rigorous dietary restrictions, resulting in a long-term, health-promoting relationship with food.

Mechanisms of Behavioural Adaptation and Coping

1. **Building Resilience:** Building resilience in the face of desire cues entails giving individuals the tools to manage urges and make nutritious choices consistently throughout time.

2. **diversified Coping Strategies:** Encouraging the use of non-food-related coping mechanisms and stress-relief strategies provides individuals with a diversified toolkit for dealing with emotional triggers and cravings in a healthy, balanced manner.

Continuous Learning and Adjustment

1. **Constant Learning and Adaptation:** A sustainable strategy includes constant learning and self-awareness, allowing individuals to modify and make educated decisions in response to changing requirements and environmental conditions.

2. **Tailored Nutrition Options:** Assisting individuals in tailoring their nutritional choices to correspond with personal preferences, cultural practices, and unique dietary needs increases long-term adherence to healthy eating habits and encourages sustainability.

Emotional and psychological health

1. **Addressing Emotional Triggers:** A sustainable approach includes comprehensive tactics for addressing emotional eating triggers

and fostering emotional resilience, laying the groundwork for a health-supportive, long-term approach to desire management.

2. Encourage Balanced Eating Habits: Fostering a balanced, non-restrictive, and non-punitive view of food and eating habits promotes a long-term, sustainable approach to cravings and dietary choices.

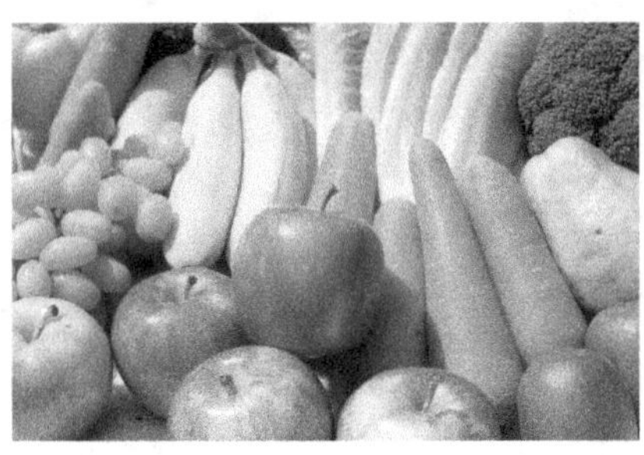

Prevention and maintenance of relapse

1. Proactive techniques: A long-term strategy emphasises the creation and implementation of relapse prevention techniques and coping mechanisms for dealing with setbacks, all of which contribute to long-term, health-promoting eating habits.

2. Reinforcement and Maintenance: Ongoing support and instruction, as well as regular reinforcement of beneficial, health-promoting behaviours, contribute to long-term commitment to balanced dietary patterns.

Change Adaptability and Flexibility

1. Environmental and Lifestyle Flexibility: A sustainable approach encourages adaptability to changing environments, schedules, and social pressures, supporting a resilient, long-term approach to desire management and healthy eating.

2. Goal Adjustment and Modification: Encouraging goal adjustment and modification in response to changing requirements and circumstances promotes a long-term, sustainable strategy to regulating urges and fostering healthy eating habits.

Individuals can create balanced eating habits and coping mechanisms that support long-term well-being by including sustainability into craving-management tactics. Sustainability entails continuing to pursue health-promoting behaviours and developing adaptable, robust techniques for regulating urges over time.

●Developing Long-Term Habits

Developing sustainable eating habits is critical for our own and the planet's health. We can lower our carbon footprint, enhance animal welfare, and improve our overall well-being by choosing conscientious food choices. Here are some comprehensive strategies to help you develop healthy eating habits:

1. **Educate Yourself:** Begin by learning about the environmental consequences of various food choices. Learn about the role of animal

husbandry on deforestation, greenhouse gas emissions, and water pollution. Investigate the advantages of plant-based diets and the significance of eating locally sourced, organic produce.

2. **Reduce Meat intake:** Reducing meat intake is one of the most effective methods to develop sustainable eating habits. Consider a flexitarian or vegetarian diet, in which you limit your meat consumption to a few days each week or eliminate it entirely. Substitute plant-based proteins for meat, such as beans, tofu, tempeh, or seitan.

3. **Select Sustainable Seafood:** If you appreciate seafood, choose selections that are responsibly sourced. Look for MSC (Marine Stewardship Council) or ASC (Aquaculture Stewardship Council) labels, which guarantee that the fish or seafood was taken or farmed in an environmentally responsible manner.

4. **Eat Local and Seasonal:** Choosing locally grown produce helps local farmers and reduces transportation emissions. Consuming seasonal fruits and vegetables maintains freshness while also reducing the need for energy-intensive greenhouse cultivation or long-distance transportation.

5. **Reduce Food Waste:** To reduce food waste, plan your meals and shop intelligently. Buy only what you need and come up with creative ways to use leftovers. Composting food leftovers instead of throwing them away minimises methane emissions.

6. **Adopt Whole Foods:** Emphasise whole foods such as fruits, vegetables, whole grains, nuts, and seeds. These meals are not only more nutritious, but they also have a smaller environmental impact than overly processed foods, which need more resources to create.

7. **Reduce packaging Waste:** To reduce waste, consider products with minimum packing or buy in bulk. When shopping or dining out, bring your own reusable bags, containers, and water bottles.

8. **Encourage Sustainable Agriculture:** Look for organic and regenerative agricultural methods that prioritise soil health, biodiversity, and water conservation. To gain access to sustainable and locally produced food, support local farmers' markets, community-supported agriculture (CSA), or join a food co-op.

9. **Grow Your Own Food:** Start a small garden or grow herbs and veggies in pots if possible. This not only gives you fresh, organic products, but it also lessens your dependency on commercially grown food.

10. **Be Aware of Water Consumption:** Conserve water by limiting your intake of water-intensive meals such as meat and dairy. Choose plant-based milk substitutes such as almond or oat milk, which require far less water to create.

Remember that developing sustainable eating habits is a journey, so make adjustments that are practical and achievable for you. Begin small, create attainable goals, and progressively add more environmentally friendly options.

●Forestalling Backslides on Food Desires / Preventing Relapses and Staying on Track

Forestalling backslides on food desires and keeping focused with your supportable dietary patterns can be testing, yet for certain techniques and mentality shifts, it is conceivable. Here are a point by point moves toward assist you with forestalling backslides and remain focused:

1. **Distinguish Triggers:** Perceive the triggers that lead to your food desires or unfortunate dietary patterns. It may very well be pressure, feelings, certain conditions, or explicit food sources. By distinguishing these triggers, you can foster methodologies to actually stay away from or oversee them.

2. **Practise Careful Eating:** Be available and completely participate in the eating experience. Focus on the taste, surface, and smell of your food. Dial back and appreciate each chomp. This training assists you with turning out to be more mindful of your body's appetite and completion signs, forestalling gorging or thoughtless eating.

3. **Prepare:** Plan your dinners and snacks ahead of time to keep away from imprudent or

unfortunate food decisions. Make a week after week dinner plan, make a staple rundown, and prep your feasts and snacks quite a bit early. Having solid choices promptly accessible lessens the possibilities of surrendering to desires.

4. **Keep Sound Snacks Convenient:** Stock your storeroom, cooler, and working environment with nutritious bites like organic products, vegetables, nuts, and seeds. At the point when desires strike, go after these better choices rather than handled or sweet tidbits. Having them promptly accessible pursues it simpler to go with manageable choices.

5. **Track down Sound Substitutes:** Recognize better substitutes for your number one liberal food sources. For instance, on the off chance that you pine for desserts, decide on regular sugars like dates or honey rather than refined sugar. On the off chance that you love seared

food varieties, have a go at baking or air broiling all things considered. Explore different avenues regarding recipes that fulfil your desires while lining up with your manageable dietary patterns.

6. **Practice Taking care of oneself:** Participate in exercises that advance taking care of oneself and lessen pressure. Stress can frequently set off desires for undesirable food varieties. Track down sound ways of overseeing pressure, like working out, contemplating, journaling, or investing energy in nature. Dealing with your general prosperity assists you with keeping focused with your reasonable dietary patterns.

7. **Look for Help:** Encircle yourself with a steady local area or look for proficient assistance if necessary. Join online gatherings or neighbourhood bunches zeroed in on economical eating or solid ways of life. Share your difficulties and victories with other people

who figure out your excursion. Consider working with a nutritionist or specialist who can give direction and responsibility.

8. **Gain from Backslides:** In the event that you truly do encounter a backslide or yield to desires, don't pummelled yourself. All things considered, use it as a potential chance to learn and develop. Think about what set off the backslide and how you can more readily deal with comparable circumstances later on. Practice self-empathy and advise yourself that misfortunes are a typical piece of the interaction.

9. **Observe Progress:** Recognize and commend your accomplishments en route. Whether it's adhering to your dinner plan for a week or effectively opposing a hankering, give yourself credit for the positive changes you're making. Compensating yourself builds up the propensity

for reasonable eating and propels you to remain focused.

10. **Remain Adaptable:** Recall that maintainable eating is a drawn out responsibility, and it's OK to be adaptable and make changes en route. Permit yourself infrequent treats or extravagances without culpability. The key is to track down an equilibrium that works for yourself and lines up with your general objectives.

By carrying out these methodologies and keeping a positive mentality, you can forestall backslides on food desires and remain focused with your practical dietary patterns. Keep in mind, it's an excursion, and each little step figures in with making a better and more maintainable way of life.

CHAPTER 7

Enabling Yourself for a Fruitful Weight Reduction Excursion

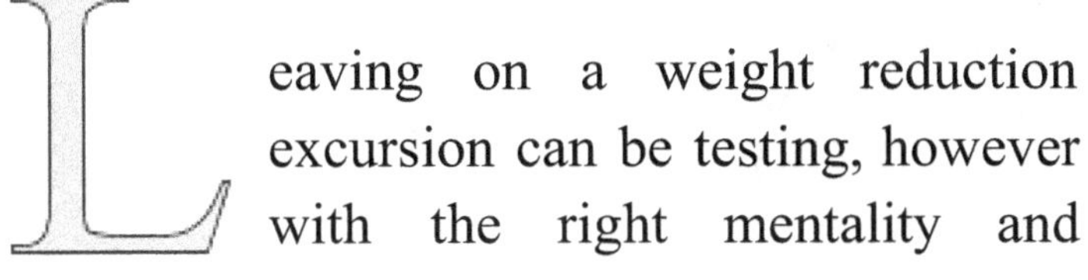

eaving on a weight reduction excursion can be testing, however with the right mentality and procedures, you can engage yourself to accomplish your objectives. Here are an itemised moves toward assist you with enabling yourself for an effective weight reduction venture:

1. **Put forth Clear and Reasonable Objectives:** Begin by defining clear and sensible objectives for your weight reduction venture. Ensure your objectives are explicit, quantifiable, attainable, important, and time-bound (Brilliant objectives).

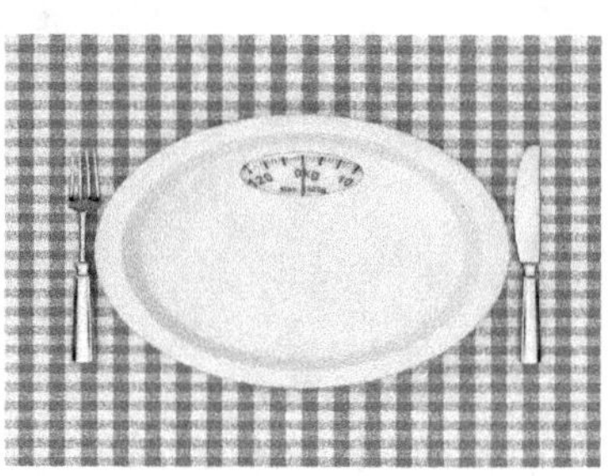

For instance, rather than saying, "I need to get more fit," put forth an objective like, "I need to shed 10 pounds in the following two months by practising for 30 minutes five times each week and following a fair dinner plan."

2. **Instruct Yourself:** Find opportunity to teach yourself about sustenance, smart dieting propensities, and exercise. Understanding how your body functions and what it needs to flourish will enable you to arrive at informed conclusions about your eating routine and way of life. Counsel trustworthy sources like enlisted dietitians or medical services experts for customised exhortation.

3. **Establish a Steady Climate:** Encircle yourself with a strong climate that empowers and spurs you on your weight reduction venture. This can incorporate joining a care group, finding a responsibility accomplice, or including your loved ones in your objectives. Having serious areas of strength for a framework will furnish you with the support and direction you really want during testing times.

4. **Practise Careful Eating:** Careful eating includes focusing on your body's craving and completion signs, as well as monitoring the taste, surface, and fulfilment of the food you eat. Dial back while eating, relish each nibble, and pay attention to your body's signs. This approach can assist you foster a better relationship with food and forestall indulging.

5. **Prepare:** Arranging your feasts and bites ahead of time can assist you with pursuing better decisions and stay away from incautious eating. Put away the opportunity every week to design your dinners, make a basic food item list, and plan sound bites. Having nutritious choices promptly accessible will make it simpler to adhere to your weight reduction plan.

6. **Consolidate Ordinary Actual work:** Customary activity is fundamental for weight reduction and generally wellbeing. Find

exercises that you appreciate and make them a piece of your everyday practice. Hold back nothing 150 minutes of moderate-power high-impact action or 75 minutes of lively force oxygen consuming movement each week, alongside strength preparing practices two times every week.

7. **Practice Taking care of oneself:** Dealing with your psychological and profound prosperity is critical during a weight reduction venture. Participate in exercises that diminish pressure, like contemplation, yoga, or investing energy in nature. Focus on taking care of oneself practices like getting sufficient rest, remaining hydrated, and overseeing feelings of anxiety to help your general wellbeing and weight reduction endeavours.

8. **Keep tabs on Your Development:** Monitor your advancement by routinely checking your weight, estimations, and body synthesis. This

can assist you with remaining spurred and recognize examples or regions where you might have to adapt. Use devices like a food journal or a wellness application to follow your dinners, exercise, and progress towards your objectives.

9. **Observe Non-Scale Triumphs:** Rather than exclusively zeroing in on the number on the scale, celebrate non-scale triumphs en route. These can incorporate expanded energy levels, further developed rest quality, squeezing into more modest dress sizes, or accomplishing wellness achievements. Perceiving and commending these accomplishments will support your certainty and keep you roused.

10. **Practice Self-Sympathy:** Be thoughtful to yourself all through your weight reduction venture. Comprehend that mishaps and difficulties are ordinary, and it's essential to show yourself empathy when things don't go

according to plan. Rather than thrashing yourself over a mistake or level, use it as a valuable chance to learn and develop.

Keep in mind, enabling yourself for a fruitful weight reduction venture requires persistence, consistency, and self-conviction. By carrying out these procedures and keeping a positive mentality, you can accomplish your weight reduction objectives and make a better and more joyful way of life.

In conclusion,

To summarise, overcoming cravings and maintaining healthy eating habits takes a combination of tactics and mindset modifications. You can prevent relapses and maintain your sustainable eating habits by identifying triggers, practising mindful eating, planning ahead, keeping healthy snacks on hand, finding healthy substitutes, practising self-care, seeking support, learning from relapses, celebrating progress, and remaining flexible.

It's critical to remember that overcoming urges is a process, and failures are typical. Instead of punishing yourself for relapses, consider them as learning opportunities to better understand your triggers and develop techniques for dealing with similar situations in the future. Self-compassion is important, as is remembering that improvement is not linear.

It is also critical to recognise your accomplishments along the route. Recognise and praise yourself for adhering to your diet, fighting temptations, or making great adjustments. This reinforces the habit of sustainable eating and inspires you to keep going.

Finally, keeping flexible and finding a workable equilibrium is essential. Allow yourself periodic sweets or indulgences without feeling guilty about it. Sustainable eating is a long-term commitment, and it's critical to establish a method of eating that fits with your overall goals and makes you happy.

You may combat cravings and stay on track with your sustainable eating habits by applying these tactics and maintaining a good mentality. Remember that every small move counts towards a healthier, more sustainable lifestyle.